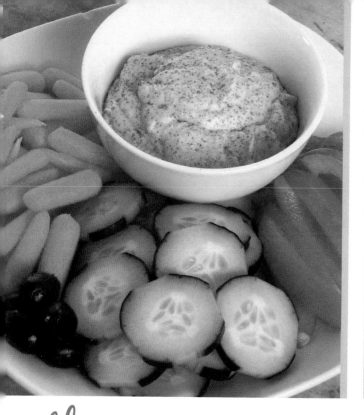

the
REAL FOOD cleanse

3 DAYS TO CLEAN UP AND RESET YOUR DIET

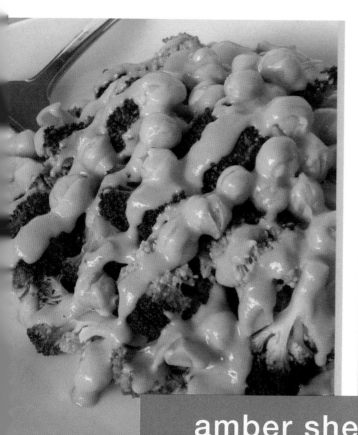
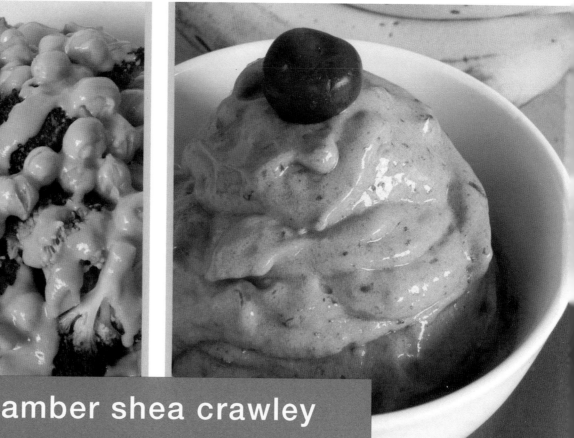

amber shea crawley

the
REAL FOOD cleanse

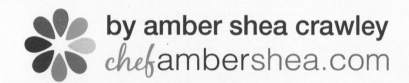

by amber shea crawley

chefambershea.com

BOOK DESIGN BY
RHIANNON DAVENPORT

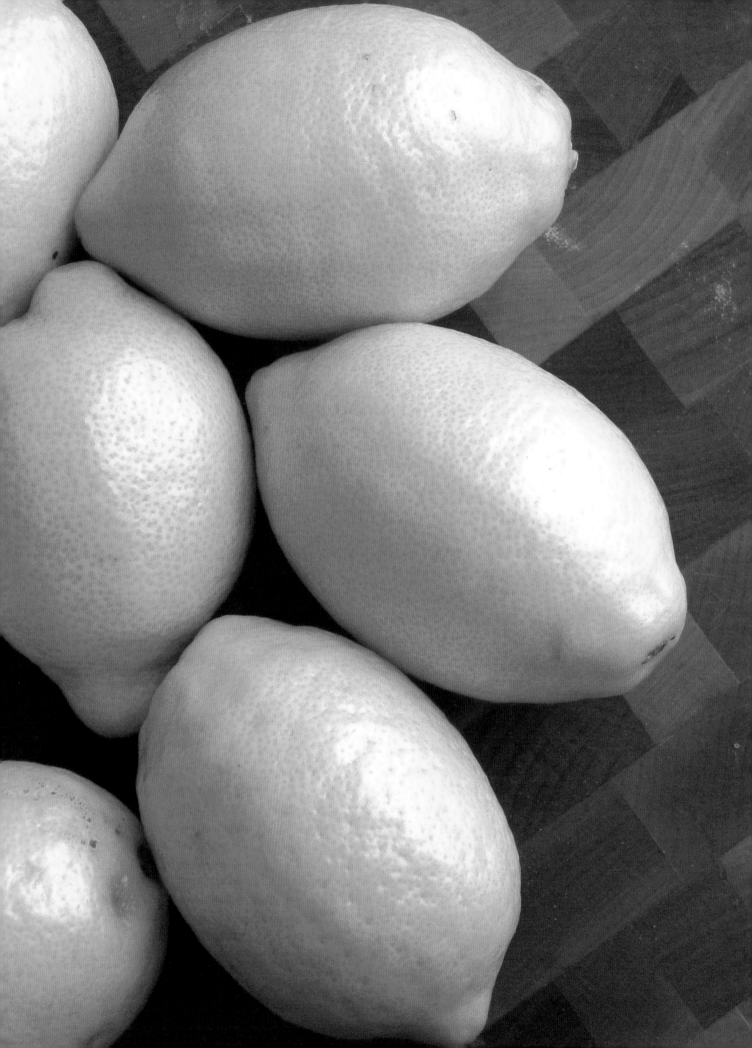

table of *contents*

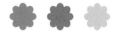

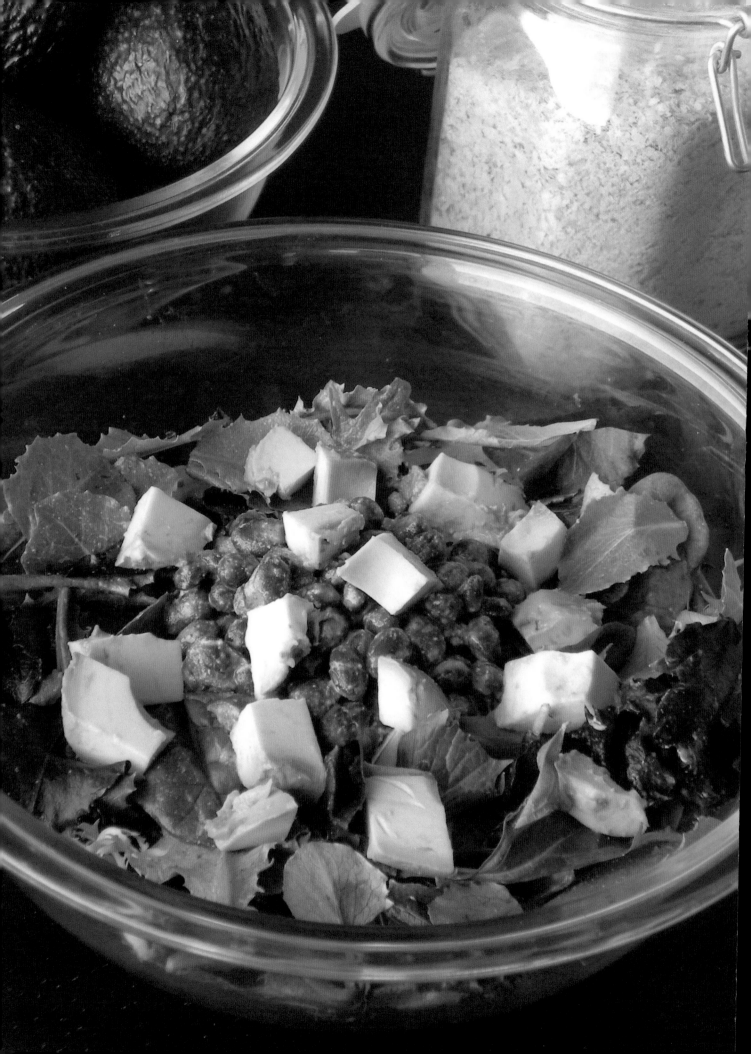

welcome to **the real food cleanse!**

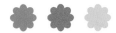

Are you ready to clean up your diet, reset your cravings, settle your digestive system, and maybe even lose a few pounds, all in just 3 days—*without* starving, juicing, or spending loads of money? The REAL FOOD Cleanse is here to help you do just that.

Everywhere you turn nowadays, you hear about radical and extreme approaches to "detoxing"—sweeping the junk out of our bodies by living for days on nothing but juice, lemonade, fruit, etc. While these methods appeal to our hope for quick fixes and magic bullets, the reality is that they can be extraordinarily difficult to complete, not to mention expensive, dull as dirt, and unlikely to result in meaningful, lasting dietary changes.

So instead, I say to you: let's cleanse on REAL FOOD! We won't feel hungry or deprived, we won't have to go buy crazy ingredients or expensive equipment, and we'll be giving our bodies ample protein, fiber, healthy fats, and micronutrients every single day.

It may sound too good to be true. You might be asking, "How can my body cleanse itself while I'm still feeding it food?" I assure you that it can and it will—our bodies are smart! To learn more about the how and why of The REAL FOOD Cleanse, read on.

what is **the real food cleanse?**

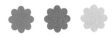

The REAL FOOD Cleanse is a 3-day diet wherein you will allow your body and cravings a chance to "reset" themselves by cutting out many heavy, pro-inflammatory, allergenic, or digestion-irritating foods. Instead, you'll eat delicious and satisfying breakfasts, lunches, dinners, and desserts filled with nutritious fruits, vegetables, seeds, and legumes. In this fashion, you'll trim calories (and, very likely, your waistline) without trimming nutrients or feeling deprived. Since you'll be eating full meals of *real food* all three days, you may be shocked at just how effortless it is to complete The REAL FOOD Cleanse!

Let's get into specifics, shall we? First, the no-no foods—here are the items you'll be saying goodbye to for the next three days:

Meat (including poultry and fish)

Dairy (milk, cheese, butter, etc.)

Eggs

Grains (and, therefore, gluten)

Soy products

Tree nuts

Oils

Caffeine (including chocolate—sorry!)

Sugar (all forms, even natural/unrefined varieties)

Artificial sweeteners

Alcohol

Instead, over your three days on The REAL FOOD Cleanse, you'll get to enjoy:

Vegetables of all kinds—green and non-green, leafy and non-leafy

Colorful and juicy fresh fruits (and a handful of dried fruit)

Fiber- and protein-rich beans

Seeds/seed butters and coconut

Cheesy, savory nutritional yeast

Green tea and/or herbal tea, if desired

It may not sound like a huge number of foods to choose from, but I promise you'll be pleasantly surprised at the variety of flavorful meals we'll craft out of such seemingly-limited ingredients. I'll make it easy, tasty, and fun!

Here are some other perks of The REAL FOOD Cleanse:

No juicer or other fancy equipment is necessary—only a food processor (or blender) is needed to prepare the recipes.

I provide you with a full shopping list that'll stock you up for all three days of the cleanse and that won't leave you with a bunch of leftover produce at the end.

No need to worry about thinking/planning ahead—I will point out every step of advance prep you need to do and when you need to do it, so there's no guesswork and no overlooking any steps.

I've built every day of the plan to be nutritionally complete in and of itself and to balance each of the other two days perfectly. Again, no guesswork!

All the recipes in the cleanse yield just a single serving, so there'll be no wasted food or leftovers lying around. That said, all recipes can also be easily doubled if you'd like to do the cleanse with your spouse or a friend!

The recipes in this cleanse are all truly simple and quick to prepare. You won't need to spend hours in the kitchen or dirty tons of dishes.

For those of you that want or need to consume a greater number of calories than what I've built into the cleanse, I've provided a "Bulk It Up" version of the plan (see page 18) that'll allow you to ratchet up the calorie count to wherever you need it to be.

By purchasing this ebook, you've also earned free access to The REAL FOOD Cleanse Facebook group. This is a private forum on Facebook where REAL FOOD Cleansers can swap tips, share ideas, ask questions, and provide each other with motivation and support. I'll be there too, moderating the board and responding to your Q's. Join us at:

http://www.facebook.com/groups/TheREALFOODCleanse/

why cleanse?

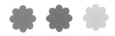

There are many reasons to do The REAL FOOD Cleanse, whether you choose to do it yearly, seasonally, monthly, or even just once.

To jump-start weight loss. I'll begin with this one, because I know it's a top interest for many people! Let's face it: making small dietary changes over time is great, and is obviously important for the long term, but it doesn't provide the same momentum and motivation that a drop on the scale can. A 3-day REAL FOOD Cleanse can give you that little boost you need to jump-start your weight loss efforts and put you on the path to your ultimate goal. It's not unusual for people to lose 3-5 pounds on this cleanse.

To reset your food cravings. If you're like me, the more junk you eat, the more junk you WANT to eat. If you've ever come to the end of a period of indulgence – such as a vacation, or the holidays, for instance – and found yourself continuing to reach for the cookies or comfort food, you could use a reset to get you back on track. A 3-day REAL FOOD Cleanse will get you back in the mindset of healthier eating.

To settle your digestion. Similarly, if you've spent a period of time indulging in junkier fare, your digestive system may be feeling the ill effects of it. If you suffer from stomachaches, heartburn, bloating, general indigestion, or constipation, a 3-day REAL FOOD Cleanse is an excellent way to give your GI tract a little TLC.

To eliminate toxins. Now, I'm not going to barrage you with any lofty ideas about toxicity, but it's a well-known fact that we're exposed to a great deal of chemicals, pollution, food additives and preservatives, and just plain processed junk on a daily basis. A cleanse can allow your body to sort through and eliminate some of these unwanted toxins.

To uncover food sensitivities. Even though you probably already know if you have a true allergy to something (although, maybe not!), you could be sensitive to certain types of food and not even know it. On a this cleanse, you'll remove potentially-irritating or difficult-to-digest foods like meat, dairy, grains, nuts, soy, and caffeine. The real value actually comes when you experiment with adding these foods back after the cleanse, if you choose—this allows you to see how they make you feel when you eat them "with a clean slate." You might decide you're better off keeping some of them out of your diet for good.

To break out of a food rut and learn some new meals. Maybe you feel stuck eating the same few things, day in and day out, but you don't feel very creative in the kitchen and don't want to go combing through dozens of cookbooks to try and come up with a meal plan. In The REAL FOOD Cleanse, I've done all the legwork for you for three full days, and you're sure to discover some new breakfasts, lunches, dinners, and desserts to freshen up your meal rotation.

Just to see what will happen. Everyone has unique reasons to want to experiment with cleansing or detoxing. Some people hope for better sleep, others for clearer skin, and still others for a happier mood. I have seen all these things happen after The REAL FOOD Cleanse, and there's a good chance they can happen for you too. There's only one way to find out!

the real food cleanse vs. *other cleanses*

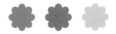

There are a great many options available to you in the world of cleansing. Here are the most popular methods, and how they stack up against The REAL FOOD Cleanse.

The Master Cleanse: Made famous by a few weight-dropping celebrities, the Master Cleanse instructs you to drink nothing but homemade lemonade (water + lemon juice + maple syrup + cayenne pepper) for TEN straight days. I'm ashamed to admit that I completed a Master Cleanse myself a few years ago, and let me just say…*never again*. Pure. Torture. And honestly, it's not at all healthy.

Juice Cleanse: Also known as a juice fast, this involves – you guessed it – drinking nothing but juice for several days (and, of course, consuming no food at all during that time). Juice fasts can be incredibly nutritious, but I can tell you from experience that they can be unbelievably hard to stick to, even for just three days—our bodies want to *eat*, to chew, to digest! Feelings of deprivation run rampant, and hunger is omnipresent. Juice fasting does get easier over time if practiced regularly, but that doesn't change the fact that a very expensive piece of equipment (a juicer—good ones cost anywhere from $150 to $450+), a significant time commitment (1 to 2 hours every morning to make the juice and clean the juicer), and a great deal of possibly-pricey produce (far more than you'd ever be able to eat) are required. There is an alternative: purchasing a 3-day juice cleanse online and having it delivered to your home. These, however, will cost you about $275 to $300 a pop. Ouch.

Green Smoothie Cleanse: As long as you have a good blender, you can cleanse by consuming nothing but green smoothies (fruit + leafy greens blended together) for a few days straight. Smoothies are much more filling than juice, and are less expensive and time-consuming to make, so a green smoothie cleanse is an easier option than a juice cleanse for busy people. However, if you're like me, you'll become bored with this option verrry quickly. After several smoothies in a row, I become cranky and start craving warm or salty or simply *chewable* food!

Mono-Fruit Cleanse: Eat unlimited amounts of a single fruit (such as bananas or watermelon), and nothing but that fruit, for a few days, and you're doing a mono-fruit ("mono" meaning "one") cleanse. The pro is that at least you get to chew something, but the big con is the same as the above: BORING! I would be so sick of fruit by the end of that cleanse, it wouldn't even be funny, so this is one I've never attempted.

Fruit and Veggie Cleanse: A classic raw-produce cleanse is an elegant and nutritious way to cleanse, albeit not terribly satisfying. Simply eat unlimited amounts of raw fruits and vegetables for 3 days—that's it! Some people can do this with ease, while others, such as myself, simply can't feel or stay full without some fat and protein in their diet. It's also just plain dull—fruit salad and crudités platters are great and all, but I need more variety in my diet to stay interested.

The REAL FOOD Cleanse: On The REAL FOOD Cleanse, you'll get to enjoy complete meals at breakfast, lunch, and dinner, and even a dessert treat each day! Some of the meals (such as the breakfasts and desserts) will be raw-food-based, while others, like dinner every night, will be hot and comforting. You'll find variety and satiety in every meal of the day, and your body will love you for it.

shopping list

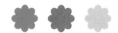

*H*ere it is: everything you'll be eating for the next three days. Just look at all the good stuff on this list! I've minimized excess, so at the end of the cleanse, almost all of this lovely food will have gone into your belly. Nom!

Fresh Produce: Fruits and veggies are the cornerstone of this cleanse, so you're going to be purchasing quite a few! I do recommend buying organic if at all possible, especially with the berries, cucumber, apple, bell pepper, and leafy greens, but if it's simply not in your budget right now, that's perfectly ok.

1 small red apple

1 lb. strawberries

½ pint (about 1 cup) blueberries

2 medium-large avocados (try and get ones that already feel ripe)

1 large bunch bananas (get ones that are as ripe as possible; 2 bunches if you'll be doing the "Bulk It Up" version of the cleanse)

1 small head garlic (optional; you will only need a couple cloves)

3 large lemons

1 large lime

1 small cucumber

1 small red bell pepper

1 small bag baby carrots

1 small sweet potato

1 small head cauliflower

1 medium head broccoli

1 small bunch kale

1 (5-oz.) bag spring mix lettuce

1 (5-oz.) bag chopped romaine lettuce

From the Bulk Bins: I like shopping at natural foods stores that have a bulk bins section. This allows me to buy small quantities of certain ingredients instead of having to invest in a big bag all at once. However, if your grocery store doesn't have bulk bins, please feel free to buy small bags of these items—I'm sure you'll find ways to use them up after the cleanse is over! If you have trouble finding things like chia seeds, ask a store manager if they carry them (sometimes they're in the supplement aisle), or order some online in advance .

Chia seeds: 2 tablespoons

Medjool dates: 6 to 8 dates

Nutritional yeast: about 1 cup

Unsweetened shredded or flaked coconut: scant ¼ cup

*Raw, shelled sunflower seeds: about ¾ cup (*ONLY if you're doing the "Bulk It Up" version of the cleanse; almonds can be substituted if you don't mind including nuts in your cleanse)

Canned/Jarred Items: If you want to be a rockstar and cook your own beans from scratch, feel free—you'll need 1½ cups each of cooked chickpeas and black beans. But for convenience, I'm calling for canned beans. I strongly recommend you try Eden brand canned beans—not only do they use BPA-free cans, they also cook their beans with kombu, a Japanese sea vegetable that helps make the beans more easily digestible (if you know what I mean).

Only two recipes in this cleanse use coconut butter, and although it's utterly delicious and you'll have no problem using it up after the cleanse, it can be expensive stuff. If you don't want to pony up for a jar, or bother making it at home (by whirring several cups of unsweetened shredded coconut from the bulk bin in your food processor for 7-10 minutes, until it achieves a smooth, buttery consistency), and you don't mind including nut products in your cleanse, you can substitute almond butter or your favorite nut butter in the two instances that coconut butter is called for. If you don't want to purchase coconut butter and you don't want to or can't include nut products in your cleanse, simply substitute additional tahini for the coconut butter.

1 (15-oz.) can chickpeas

1 (15-oz.) can black beans

1 small jar or can olives (Kalamata or your favorite variety)

1 jar tahini, a.k.a. sesame seed butter (raw or roasted—I prefer the flavor of roasted)

1 small jar coconut butter (or your favorite nut butter, such as almond butter)

Frozen Foods: If it's summer and/or fresh cherries are in season where you are, feel free to use those instead! I opt for frozen because they're more widely available and convenient.

1 (10-oz.) bag frozen sweet cherries (check the label to make sure there's no sugar added)

Pantry Staples: Before you go grocery shopping for the cleanse, make sure you have the following items in your pantry, and if not, make sure to pick some up at the store.

Ground cinnamon

Curry powder

Chili powder

Ground cumin

Sea salt

Prepared yellow mustard

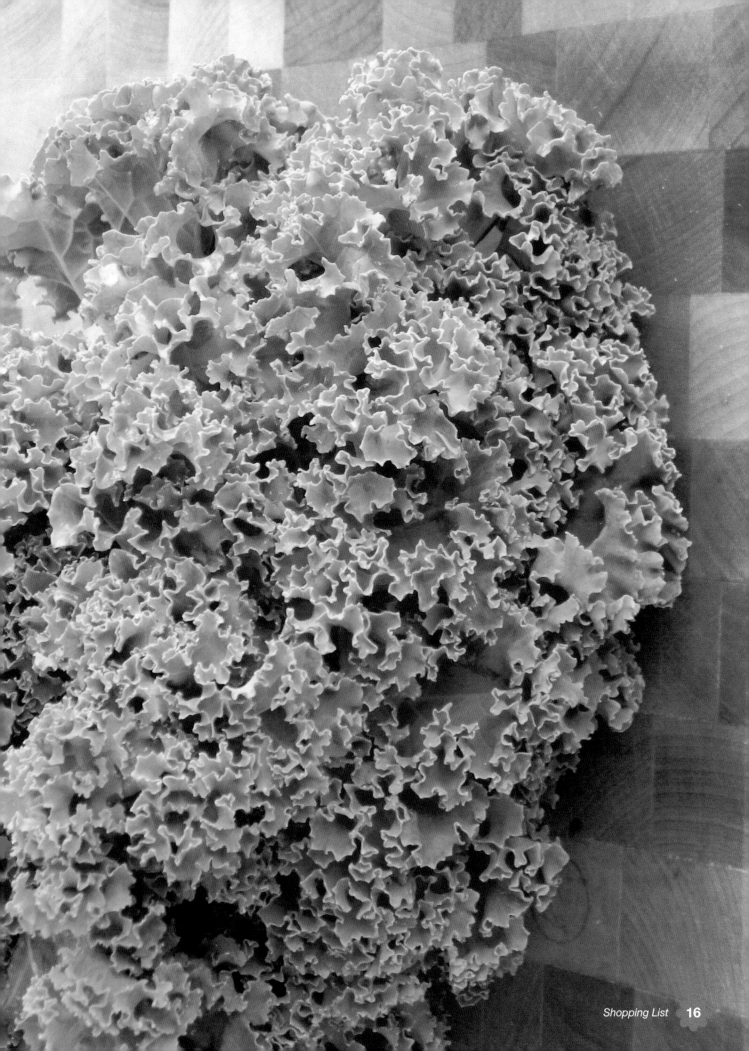

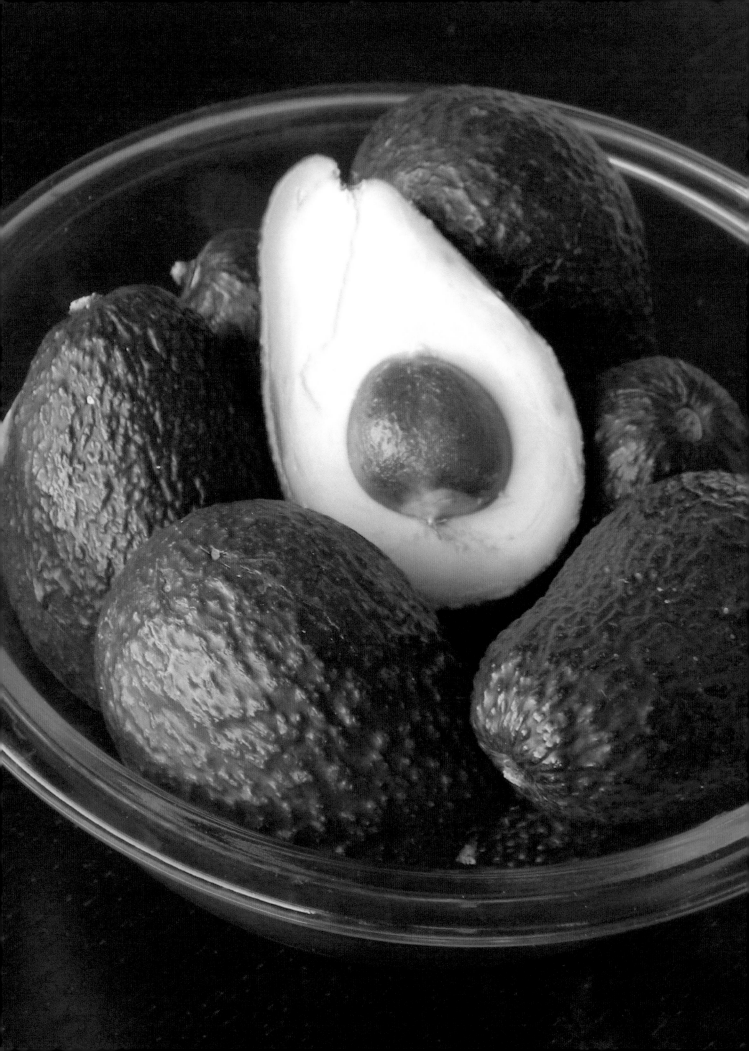

the "bulk it up" plan

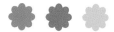

For those of you that will want or need to consume a greater number of calories than what I've built into the plan, I created the "Bulk It Up" version of The REAL FOOD Cleanse. This will allow you to ratchet up the calorie count of the cleanse to wherever you need it to be.

Who should do the "Bulk It Up" version of the plan?

Men over 5'4" tall

Women over 5'10" tall

Anyone with a physically active job or daily routine

Anyone who plans on doing strenuous or high-intensity exercise during the cleanse

The "Bulk It Up" plan is super-simple to implement. Here's how it works:

- To each day of the cleanse, add ¼ **cup raw sunflower seeds** (or almonds) and **1 ripe banana**. You may either add these to the meals – for example, sprinkle the seeds on your salad at lunch and eat the banana with your breakfast – or you may eat them as snacks (together, as a single snack, or separately, as two snacks). This will add 300 calories to your cleanse each day, bringing your daily intake to 1700-1750 calories.

- To add more calories beyond this, add **additional ripe bananas** (up to 3 per day). Each banana will add about 100 more calories to your cleanse.

In this way, you have options to add 300, 400, 500, or 600 calories to each day of the meal plan, bringing the total daily calories as high as about 2,000, if you so choose. The only reason I cap it out at 2,000 is that this is still meant to be a cleanse, so keeping food intake semi-light is part of the point. That said, by all means please add the calories if you are particularly active, have a medical need for more calories, or simply find yourself too hungry with the meal plan as given.

preparing for the cleanse

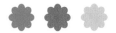

Arre you ready and rarin' to go?! As promised, I've got all your advance preparation steps already considered and covered, so you just have to read and follow along. The following are my recommendations for how and when to prepare for the cleanse.

3 to 5 days before the cleanse:

Reduce your consumption of meat, dairy, coffee, and sugar.

If you're out and can run by a grocery store, go ahead and buy your 2 avocados and 1-2 bunches of bananas now so they can get nice and ripe. (If this isn't convenient for you, no big deal.)

1 to 3 days before the cleanse:

- Reduce even further – or, better yet, eliminate altogether – your meat, dairy, coffee, and sugar intake.

- Read this entire ebook, cover to cover, if you haven't already. It's great mental preparation for you, and can make you feel excited about what's to come!

1 to 2 days before the cleanse:

- Go shopping! Print out the shopping list and take it (and a pen) to the store with you so you don't forget anything. Remember, if you didn't buy avocados and bananas earlier in the week, to try and look for already-ripe ones if at all possible.

The Night Before Day 1

Completing these preparatory tasks the night before the cleanse will make your life a lot easier, especially if you have hectic mornings and/or have a job to commute to. Each day of the cleanse, I'll give you a list like this of what to do to prepare for the following day. This may seem like a lot, but keep in mind you're basically pre-making your whole breakfast and lunch for the next day. If you work from home or it's a weekend, you can skip these preparations and simply make each meal fresh.

Squeeze the juice from your lemons and limes (separately!) and strain out any seeds. Store the juices in two glass jars or containers in the refrigerator. Use throughout the cleanse whenever lemon or lime juice is called for in a recipe.

Hull and slice 1½ cups of strawberries (about half the 1-lb. container you bought) for your breakfast in the morning; place them in a large bowl or container. Core and chop the apple for breakfast and add it to the container with the strawberries. Add a couple teaspoons of lemon juice, put the lid on, shake it up, and place it in the fridge till the morning. (*This is optional—you can prep this fresh in the morning if you have the time.)

Make the dressing for tomorrow's lunchtime salad by combining 2 tablespoons nutritional yeast, 2 tablespoons lime juice, 1 tablespoon tahini, 1 tablespoon water, ½ teaspoon chili powder, ½ teaspoon ground cumin, and ¼ teaspoon sea salt in a small glass jar or container. Put the lid on, shake vigorously to mix, and place it in the fridge till lunch tomorrow.

Open the can of black beans, pour them into a strainer set over the sink, and rinse and drain them thoroughly. Divide them evenly between two containers (about ¾ cup per container) and place both containers in the fridge.

Open the 5-oz. bag of spring mix lettuce and transfer about 1½ cups (a couple handfuls) to a small baggie or container; close and place in the fridge. Transfer the remaining spring mix into a large container, put on the lid, and place in the fridge.

Cut one ripe avocado in half (leaving the pit IN and the peel on). Sprinkle about a half-teaspoon of lemon juice over each half and rub it across the surface with your finger. Wrap each half very snugly and securely in plastic wrap and place both halves in the fridge.

Now your lunch for tomorrow is ready to go, if it's a weekday and you'll need to take it to work. Go ahead and cluster these components together in a section of your fridge so you can grab them all and get going tomorrow morning:

The large container of spring mix lettuce

One of the containers of black beans

One half of the cut avocado (I recommend grabbing the half *without* the pit, as the half with the pit will last longer)

The jar/container of dressing

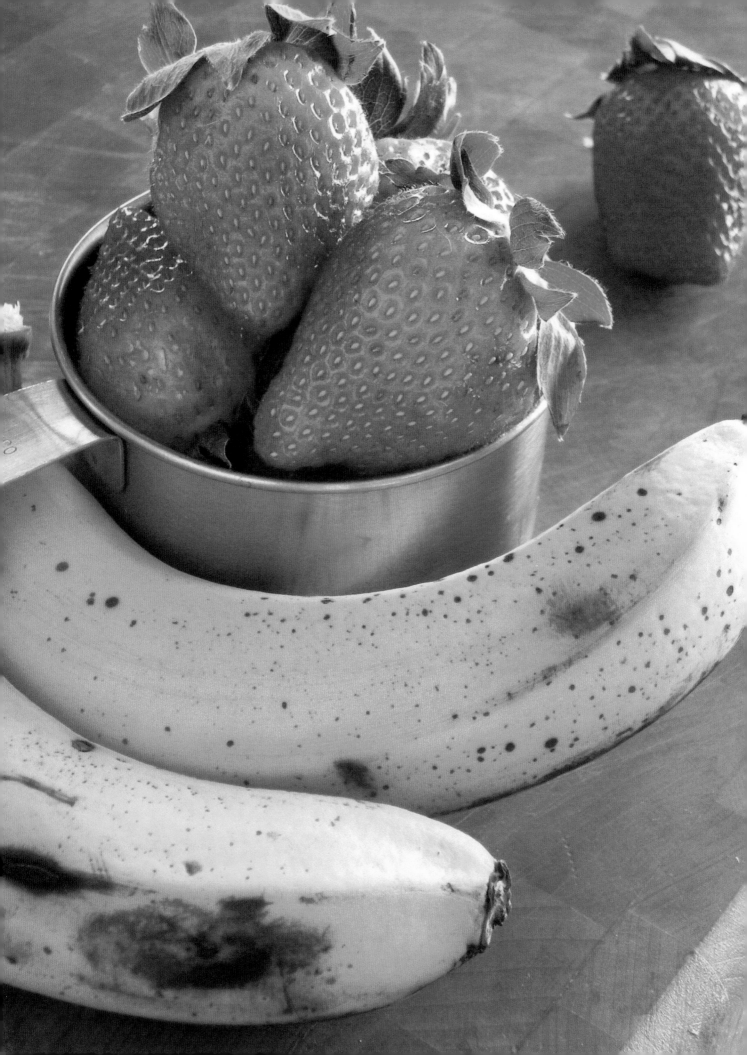

day one

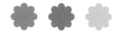

elcome to Day 1 of The REAL FOOD Cleanse! If you completed last night's list of prep steps for today, it should be smooth sailing for you this morning and afternoon. Don't be nervous—this will be easier than you think.

Here's what you have to look forward to today:

Day One Menu

Breakfast Strawberry Blonde Breakfast Bowl

Lunch Zingy Spring Mix Salad with Black Beans

Dinner Cheese-Smothered Broccoli & Chickpeas

Dessert Buttery Stuffed Dates with Berries

The Strawberry Blonde Breakfast Bowl is a blushing beauty of a b-fast that'll start your day off right, with four whole servings of fruit. The Zingy Spring Mix Salad with Black Beans will really fill you up at lunch and carry you through the afternoon, thanks to its abundance of beans and its healthy-fat-filled avocado topping. If you like comfort food even a little, you will fall hard for the Cheese-Smothered Broccoli & Chickpeas at dinner—ooh, baby! And as if that weren't enough, you'll end the day with Buttery Stuffed Dates with Berries, a candy-like treat that you'll hardly believe is cleanse-friendly and healthy for you.

Nutritionally, we're packing hefty amounts of protein and fiber into day 1 so that the sudden drop in calories doesn't shock your body too much.

Nutritional Totals for Day 1:
1414 calories | 55 grams fat | 216 grams carbohydrates
58 grams fiber | 53 grams protein | 993 milligrams sodium

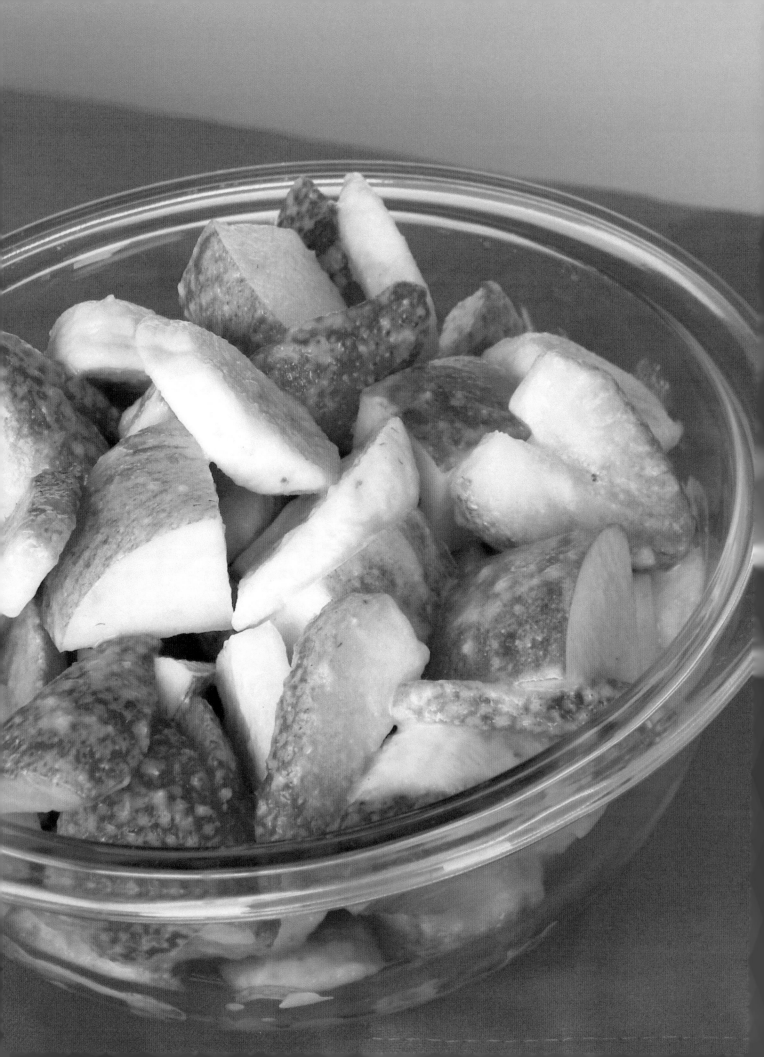

Strawberry Blonde Breakfast Bowl

This may look like a ton of fruit, but I suspect you'll plow through it quickly and gleefully. Having it in fruit salad form like this – such that you have to chew it – will help keep you full longer than if you were to blend it up as a smoothie. Feel free to use coconut butter (or even almond butter, if you don't mind including nuts in your cleanse) in place of the tahini if you prefer; just make sure to combine it with room-temperature (not cold) water so it doesn't immediately solidify.

1 tablespoon tahini
1½ tablespoons water
1½ cups fresh strawberries (½ of the 1-lb. box), hulled and sliced

1 small red apple, cored and diced
1 medium ripe banana, peeled and sliced
Ground cinnamon, for sprinkling (optional)

In a medium bowl, use a fork to stir the tahini and water together until smooth.

If you chopped your strawberries and apple last night, take them out of the fridge and add them to the bowl with the tahini mixture. If you didn't, chop them now and add them to the bowl. Peel and slice the banana and add it to the bowl as well.

Toss and stir the fruit to coat it with the tahini "dressing." Sprinkle with cinnamon, if desired, and serve immediately.

Nutritional Information:
302 calories, 9.6 grams fat, 56.3 grams carbs, 5.1 grams protein

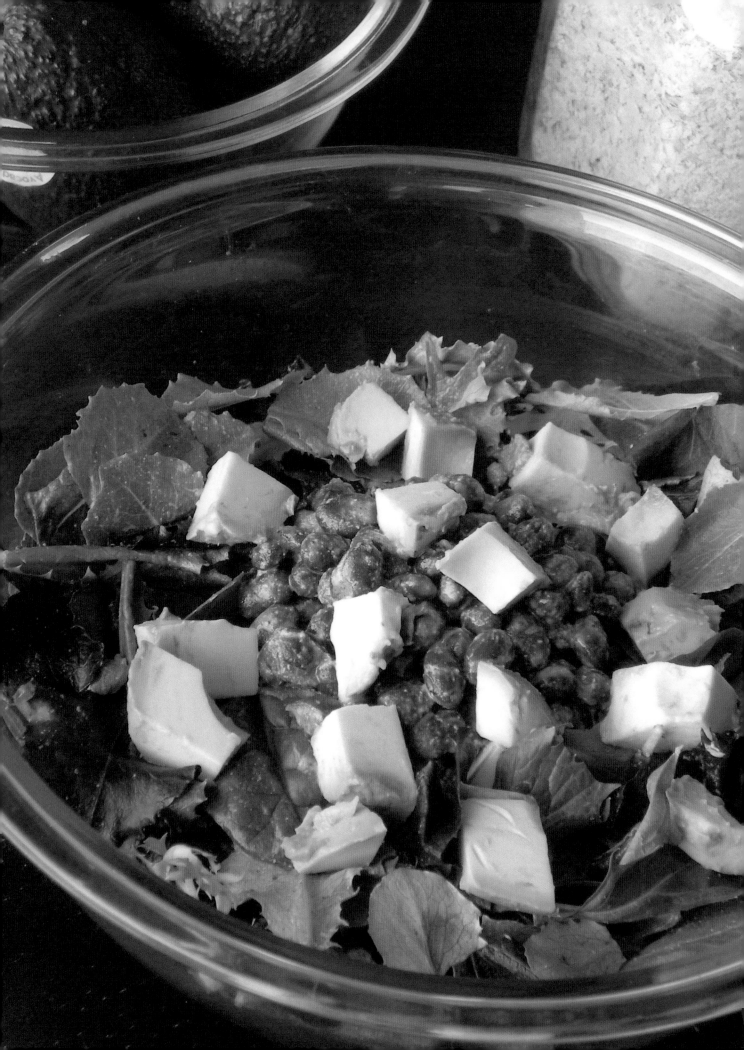

Zingy Spring Mix Salad with Black Beans

This Mexican-inspired, ultra-filling salad has it all: protein- and fiber-rich beans, healthy monounsaturated fats from the avocado, loads of minerals and chlorophyll in the leafy greens, and a creamy, cheesy, zippy lime juice dressing to pull it all together. It's sure to keep you more than satisfied until dinnertime rolls around.

2 tablespoons nutritional yeast
2 tablespoons lime juice
1 tablespoon tahini
1 tablespoon water
½ teaspoon chili powder
½ teaspoon ground cumin

¼ teaspoon sea salt
¾ cup (½ of the 15-oz. can) black beans, rinsed
   and drained
1 (5-oz.) bag spring mix (reserve about 1½ cups
   for dinner tomorrow)
½ large ripe avocado, pitted, peeled, and diced

If you already prepared and set aside all the components last night, skip to step 6.

If you did not already prepare the dressing last night, combine the nutritional yeast, lime juice, tahini, water, chili powder, ground cumin, and sea salt in a small bowl and whisk together.

Open the 5-oz. bag of spring mix lettuce and transfer about 1½ cups (a couple handfuls) to a small baggie or container; close and place in the fridge for tomorrow's dinner. Transfer the remaining spring mix into a large bowl.

Open the can of black beans, pour them into a strainer set over the sink, and rinse and drain them thoroughly. Measure out about ¾ cup (about half the total amount), transfer it to a small container, put on the lid, and refrigerate it for tomorrow's dinner. You should have about ¾ cup of beans remaining in the strainer.

Cut one ripe avocado in half. Sprinkle about a half-teaspoon of lemon juice over the half with the pit and rub it across the surface with your finger, then wrap this half very snugly and securely in plastic wrap and place it in the fridge for tomorrow's dessert.

Scoop the flesh out of the [other] avocado half and dice it up.

Pour two tablespoons of the dressing over the spring mix lettuce and toss lightly to combine it and coat the leaves. Scoop the black beans on top of the lettuce and drizzle the remaining dressing on top. (You can also pre-toss the remaining dressing with the black beans before adding them to the salad.) Scatter the diced avocado on top, and enjoy immediately.

Nutritional Information:
437 calories, 20.5 grams fat, 49.6 grams carbs, 20.3 grams protein

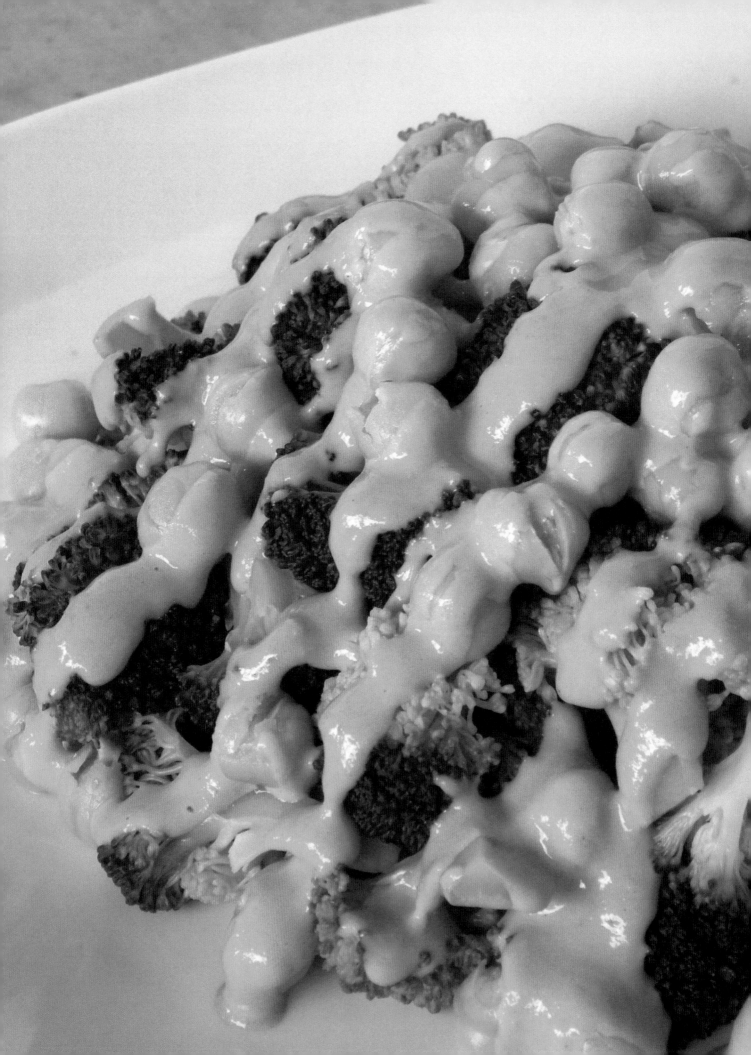

Cheese-Smothered Broccoli & Chickpeas

File this one straight under "I can't believe it's healthy," let alone cleanse-friendly! Just wait till you taste this salty, tangy, savory cheese sauce. I made the serving size nice and generous, so enjoy every bite! Steaming the broccoli first helps soften its difficult-to-digest cellulose fibers.

1 medium head broccoli, cut into florets
½ cup (one-third of a 15-oz. can) chickpeas, rinsed and drained
¼ cup nutritional yeast
2½ tablespoons water
1½ tablespoons tahini

1 tablespoon lemon juice
½ teaspoon prepared yellow mustard
¼ teaspoon sea salt

Bring an inch of water to a simmer in a stockpot over medium heat and fit a metal steamer into the pot. If you don't own a steamer, bring 6 cups of water to a boil in a stockpot or teapot.

Cut the head of broccoli into small florets. (Discard the large stem, or wrap it in tinfoil and freeze it to make vegetable broth someday.) Place the florets into the steamer and fit the lid tightly onto the stockpot. If not steaming, place the florets in a large bowl and pour the 6 cups of boiling water over the broccoli.

Open the can of chickpeas, pour them into a strainer set over the sink, and rinse and drain them thoroughly. Measure out about 1 cup, transfer it to a small container, put on the lid, and refrigerate it for later in the cleanse. You should have about ½ cup of chickpeas remaining in the strainer; add these to the steamer or the hot water with the broccoli.

In a small bowl, combine the nutritional yeast, water, tahini, lemon juice, mustard, and salt and whisk with a fork until smooth.

If you're steaming the broccoli, allow it to steam for 5 to 7 minutes total, until fork-tender. If you poured boiling water over it, let it sit just until you finish with the beans and cheese sauce, then carefully pour it into a strainer and shake all the water off.

Transfer the steamed or blanched broccoli and chickpeas to a large bowl or plate. Spoon the cheese sauce all over it and serve immediately.

Nutritional Information:
392 calories, 15.6 grams fat, 47.6 grams carbs, 25.2 grams protein

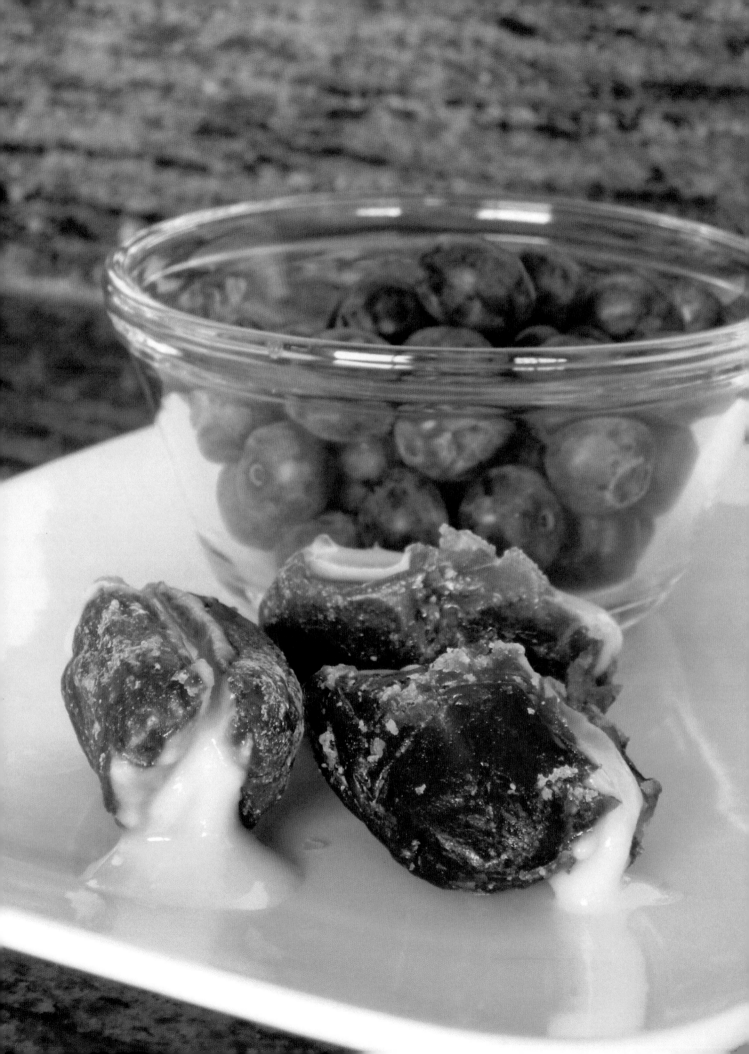

Buttery Stuffed Dates with Berries

Funky-looking? Sure. Delicious? Oh, hell yes. Dates stuffed with "butter" (coconut butter, in this case, though you can use to tahini if you prefer, or even almond or cashew butter if you don't mind including nuts in your cleanse) practically taste like candy! A handful of juicy fresh berries on the side helps to complement the concentrated richness of the dates and coconut.

3 soft Medjool dates
1 tablespoon coconut butter, softened
¼ cup fresh blueberries

Cut slits in the sides of your Medjool dates and remove the pits, but keep the dates whole (don't tear them in half/into pieces).

Spoon 1 teaspoon coconut butter into each date.

You can either squeeze a couple blueberries inside each date as well, or enjoy them on the side.

Serve immediately.

Nutritional Information:
312 calories, 9.3 grams fat, 62.4 grams carbs, 2.5 grams protein

before going to bed **at the end of day 1**

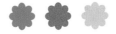

Open the bag of frozen cherries and divide them evenly between two containers. Place one container back in the freezer and place the other container in the fridge to thaw overnight.

Make the hummus for tomorrow's lunch by placing 2/3 cup of the refrigerated chickpeas into the food processor. (You should have about 1/3 cup chickpeas remaining; leave those in the container and put them back in the refrigerator for dinner on day 3.) Add 2 tablespoons nutritional yeast, 2 tablespoons lemon juice, 2 tablespoons water, 1 tablespoon tahini, 1 small clove minced garlic (if desired), and a scant ¼ teaspoon sea salt to the food processor and pulse or purée until smooth (or leave it somewhat chunky, if desired), adding another tablespoon of water if needed. Transfer the hummus to a container and place in the refrigerator.

Slice the cucumber and place the slices in a large container. Seed and slice the red bell pepper and add to the same container. Open the bag of baby carrots and measure out ¾ cup; place these in the same container. (Wrap up the remaining baby carrots and store them in the fridge—these can be emergency snacks for any point in the cleanse.) Open the jar of olives and add a handful to the container of veggies, if desired. Put a lid on the container of veggies and refrigerate it for tomorrow's lunch.

Now your lunch for tomorrow is ready to go, if it's a weekday and you'll need to take it to work. Go ahead and cluster these components together in a section of your fridge so you can grab them both and get going tomorrow morning:

    The container of cut mixed vegetables

    The container of hummus

day *two*

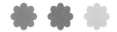

Welcome to Day 2 of The REAL FOOD Cleanse! How did you do yesterday? Were you surprised by how full you felt after those meals? Were you pleased with the portion sizes? Did you experience any digestive discomfort, or did your system handle the diet change smoothly? How did you sleep last night? Take a moment this morning to "check in" with your body and see how you're feeling. It's only been one day, so don't expect miracles, but maybe you woke up today with a little extra spring in your step.

Here's what's on tap for today:

Day Two Menu

Breakfast Chilly Cherry-Coconut Porridge

Lunch Mediterranean Mezze Platter with One-Minute Hummus

Dinner Fiesta Black Beans with Coconut-Buttered Sweet Potato

Dessert Strawberry Avocado Pudding

The Chilly Cherry-Coconut Porridge is like a chunky, antioxidant-rich smoothie you get to eat with a spoon—a "spoonie," if you will! The Mediterranean Mezze Platter with One-Minute Hummus at lunch offers you a buffet of fresh, crisp veggies to dip in a quick-to-whip-up hummus. Dinnertime's Fiesta Black Beans with Coconut-Buttered Sweet Potato is a huge, hot plate of deliciousness, and you'll get to enjoy a giant bowl of sweet-tart Strawberry Avocado Pudding for dessert.

Nutritionally, after yesterday's ample doses of protein and fat (which helped ease your transition to a lower calorie intake), we're lightening up a bit on those macronutrients today and giving you more energy-boosting fruit and vegetable carbohydrates instead.

Nutritional Totals for Day 2:
1438 calories | 43 grams fat | 240 grams carbohydrates
49 grams fiber | 42 grams protein | 783 milligrams sodium

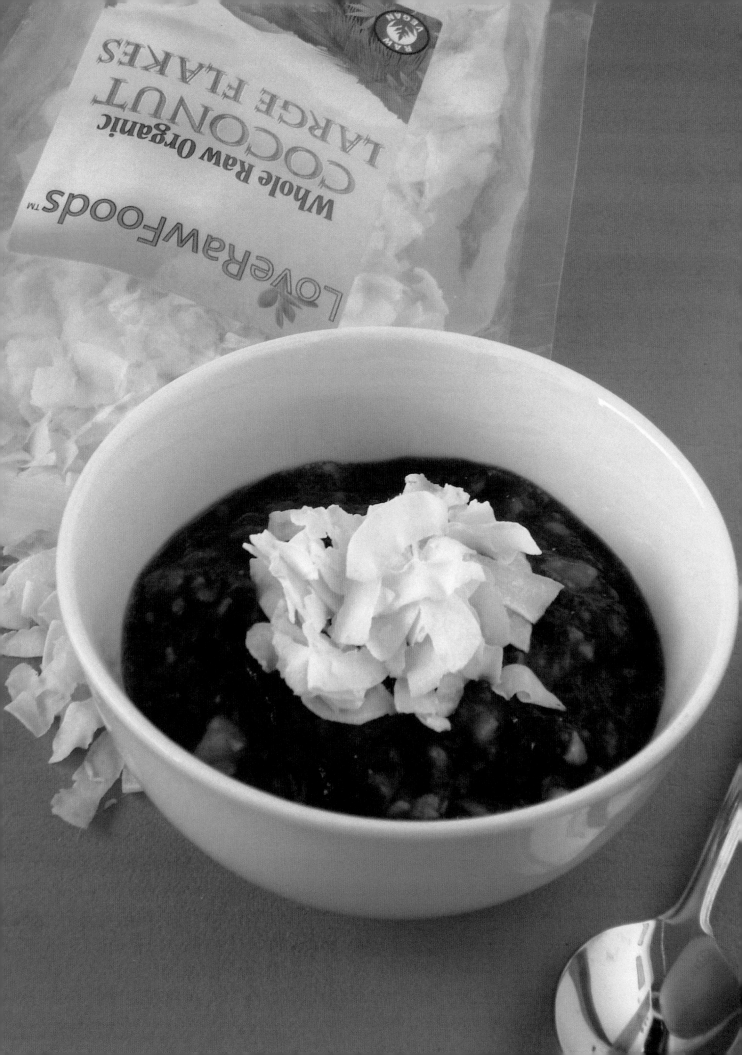

Chilly Cherry-Coconut Porridge

The coconut adds chewiness and healthy, satisfying fats to this fruity breakfast bowl. If the cherries and banana don't create enough natural sweetness for you, pulse or stir one pitted, minced Medjool date into the mixture.

½ (10-oz.) bag frozen cherries, thawed in the
    refrigerator overnight
1 small (or ½ large) ripe banana, peeled
    and sliced
2 tablespoons unsweetened shredded (or 3
    tablespoons flaked) coconut
Ground cinnamon, for sprinkling (optional)

Remove the thawed frozen cherries from the refrigerator and place in the bowl of a food processor (a mini [3- or 4-cup] processor works especially well here). Peel and slice or break the ripe banana into chunks and add it to the food processor with the cherries.

Pulse the fruit together until the mixture is chunky and just combined (do not purée it). Transfer to a bowl and sprinkle the coconut on top.

Dust with cinnamon, if desired, and serve immediately.

Nutritional Information:
289 calories, 8 grams fat, 53.5 grams carbs, 1.4 grams protein

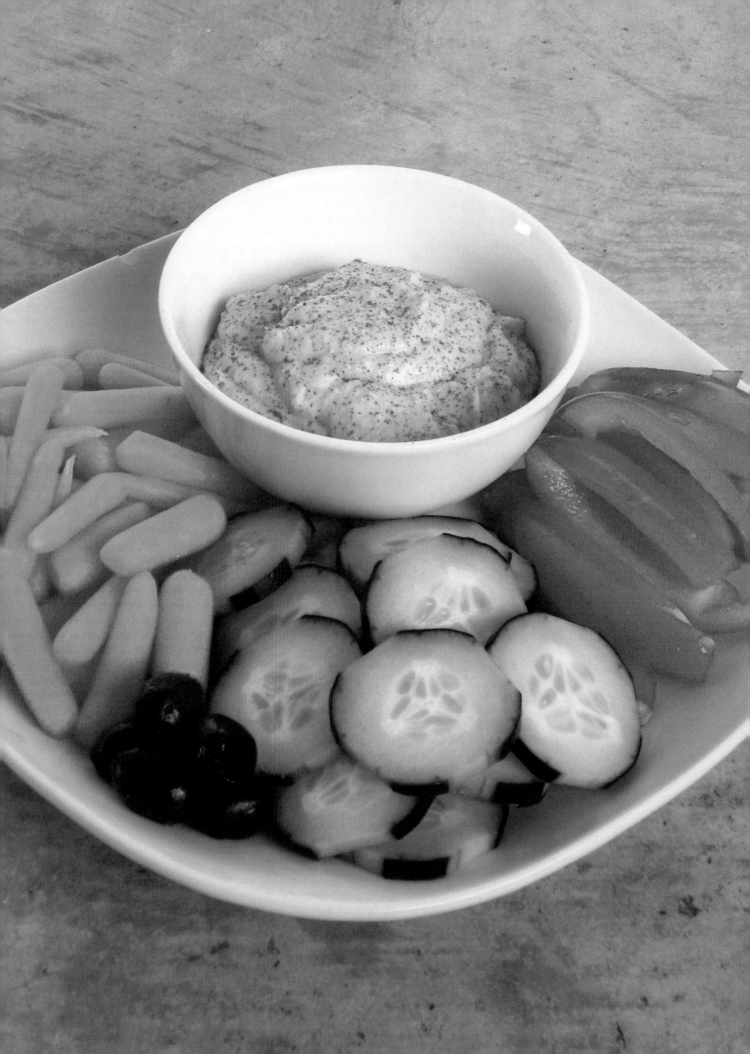

Mediterranean Mezze Platter with One-Minute Hummus

Now this is my kind of finger food! A mountain of fresh, crisp raw crudités awaits you, ready to dip into a homemade hummus you can put together in seconds flat.

2/3 cup chickpeas, rinsed and drained
2 tablespoons nutritional yeast
2 tablespoons lemon juice
2 to 3 tablespoons water
1 tablespoon tahini
1 small (or ½ large) clove garlic, peeled and
   minced (optional)

Scant ¼ teaspoon sea salt
1 small cucumber, sliced
1 small red bell pepper, seeded and sliced
¾ cup baby carrots
Handful of Kalamata olives (optional)

If you already prepared all the components of this meal last night, skip to step 4.

If you didn't already make the hummus last night, place 2/3 cup of the refrigerated chickpeas into the food processor. (You should have about 1/3 cup chickpeas remaining; leave those in the container and put them back in the refrigerator for dinner on day 3.) Add the nutritional yeast, lemon juice, 2 tablespoons water, tahini, garlic (if desired), and sea salt to the food processor and pulse or purée until smooth (or leave it somewhat chunky, if desired), adding another tablespoon of water if needed. Transfer the hummus to a small bowl.

If you didn't already prep the veggies last night, slice the cucumber and place the slices on a large plate. Seed and slice the red bell pepper and add to the same plate. Open the bag of baby carrots and measure out ¾ cup; place these on the same plate. (Wrap up the remaining baby carrots and store them in the fridge—these can be emergency snacks for any point in the cleanse.) Open the jar of olives and add a handful to the veggie plate, if desired.

Serve immediately, dipping the veggies into the hummus (healthy finger food!) or using a spoon to scoop the hummus on top of the veggies.

Nutritional Information:
395 calories, 12.2 grams fat, 58.2 grams carbs, 18.8 grams protein

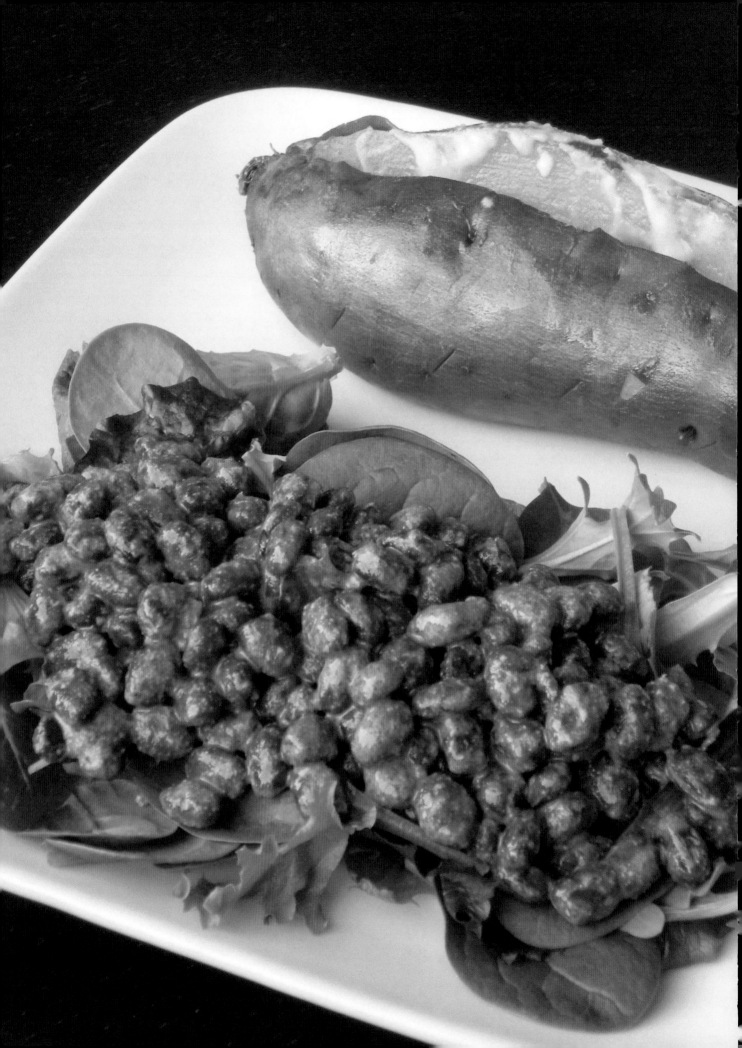

Fiesta Black Beans with Coconut-Buttered Sweet Potato

This supper of zesty seasoned black beans, a healthy handful of leafy greens, and a tender baked sweet potato slathered with creamy coconut butter creates a comforting combo that'll delight taste buds and tummies alike.

1 small sweet potato
2 tablespoons nutritional yeast
1 tablespoon lime juice
½ teaspoon chili powder
½ teaspoon ground cumin
1/8 teaspoon sea salt

¾ cup black beans (reserved from yesterday's lunch), rinsed and drained
1½ cups spring mix lettuce (reserved from yesterday's lunch)
1 tablespoon coconut butter, softened
Ground cinnamon, for sprinkling (optional)

At least an hour before dinner, preheat the oven to 400°F.

Poke the sweet potato with a fork in several places, then wrap it tightly in a sheet of tinfoil and place it on a baking sheet. When the oven is preheated, place the baking sheet in the oven and bake for 45 minutes, flipping the wrapped potato over with tongs halfway through.

Remove the container with the remaining ¾ cup of black beans from the fridge. Add the nutritional yeast, lime juice, chili powder, cumin, and salt, put the lid back on, and shake well to combine. Set aside until the potato is done baking.

When the timer goes off, make sure the potato can be pierced easily all the way through with a butter knife—if so, it's thoroughly baked. (If not, rewrap it and bake it for 10-15 more minutes.) Remove the baking sheet from the oven and set it aside to allow the potato to cool slightly.

Warm the seasoned beans in a small saucepan on the stove over medium heat. (You may warm them in the microwave instead if you choose, though I always recommend using the stove.)

To serve, pile the reserved 1½ cups spring mix lettuce onto half of a large plate. Scoop or spoon the warm seasoned beans on top. Carefully remove the baked sweet potato from the tinfoil, use a knife to cut a slit from one end to the other (cut all the way through the inside flesh of the potato, but don't slice through the bottom), and transfer it to the plate next to the beans. Spoon the tablespoon of coconut butter inside the cut sweet potato, sprinkle with a bit of cinnamon if desired, and serve.

Nutritional Information:
436 calories, 10.6 grams fat, 71.1 grams carbs, 18.1 grams protein

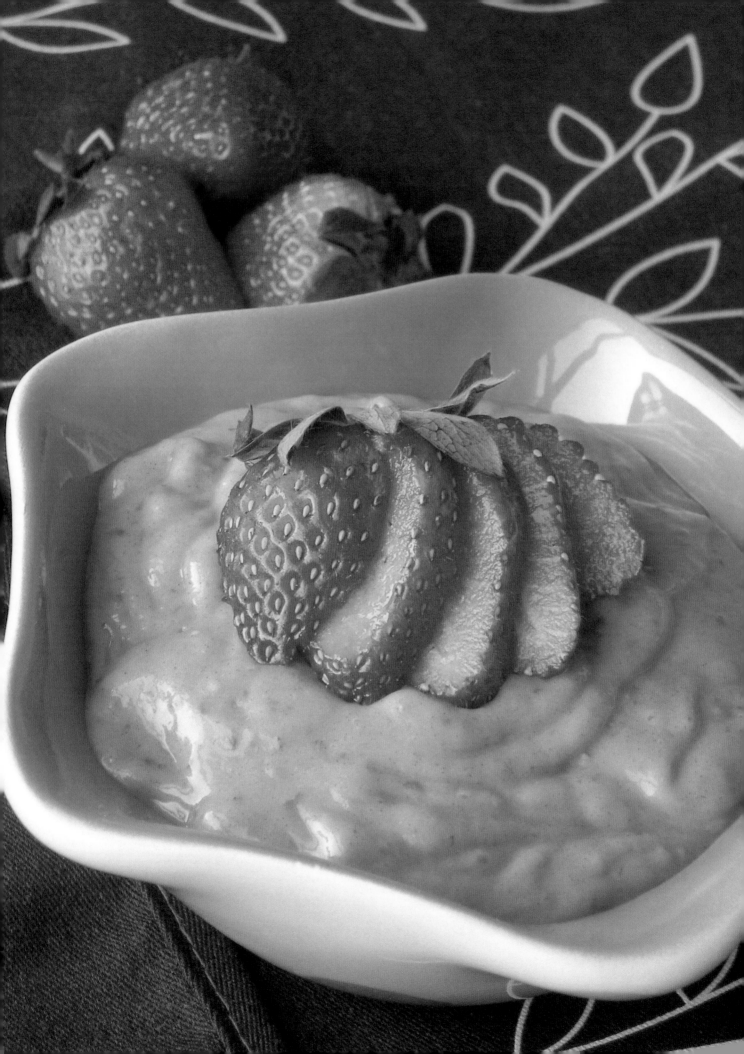

Strawberry Avocado Pudding

It may sound like an odd pairing, but don't knock it till you try it! This cleansing pudding is packed with fiber, vitamin C, and monounsaturated fats. If you feel your strawberries don't add enough natural sweetness (off-season strawberries can be a little tart sometimes), you can blend in an extra pitted date or two.

2 large Medjool dates, pitted and soaked in ¼
    cup hot water for 10-20 minutes
½ large ripe avocado, pitted, peeled, and diced
1½ cups fresh strawberries (the remainder of the
    1-lb. box), hulled and sliced
1 teaspoon fresh lemon juice
Pinch of sea salt

Place the pitted dates in a small bowl and add about ¼ cup very hot water. Set aside for at least 10 minutes to allow the dates to soften. Meanwhile, hull and slice the strawberries.
Grab the other half of yesterday's avocado from the fridge and take it out of the plastic wrap. Remove and discard the pit. Scoop the avocado out of its skin and into the food processor (or a blender).
Add the strawberries, lemon juice, and salt and pulse to combine.
Remove the softened dates from the hot water (do not discard the soaking water) and add them to the food processor as well. Blend the mixture together until it is smooth and combined. You can add the soaking water from the dates, about a teaspoon at a time, only if needed to help the mixture blend. Transfer the pudding to a bowl and serve immediately.

Nutritional Information:
317 calories, 12.1 grams fat, 57 grams carbs, 3.7 grams protein

before going to bed at the end of day 2

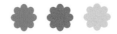

Combine 2 tablespoons chia seeds and 2/3 cup lukewarm water in a medium bowl or container and stir together. Cover and place in the refrigerator overnight.

Peel 2 small (or 1½ large) ripe bananas and cut or break them into thick slices. Place the slices on a piece of waxed paper (set the waxed paper on a plate, if desired) and transfer to the freezer to freeze overnight.

Make the dressing for tomorrow's lunchtime salad by combining 1 medium ripe avocado (pitted, peeled, and chopped), 3 tablespoons water, 2 tablespoons nutritional yeast, 2 tablespoons lemon juice, 1 clove minced garlic (if desired), and ¼ teaspoon sea salt in a food processor (a mini processor works well here). Blend until completely smooth, adding another tablespoon of water if needed. Transfer to a small jar or container and place it in the fridge till lunch tomorrow.

Coarsely chop ¼ cup Kalamata olives, transfer to a small jar or container, and place in the fridge till lunch tomorrow.

Now your lunch for tomorrow is ready to go, if it's a weekday and you'll need to take it to work. Go ahead and cluster these components together in a section of your fridge so you can grab them all and get going tomorrow morning:

>   The bag of romaine lettuce (plus a vessel to eat the salad out of, if necessary!)

>   The jar/container of avocado dressing

>   The jar/container of chopped olives

day three

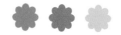

You've made it to Day 3 of The REAL FOOD Cleanse! You're in the home stretch now. It may not feel very challenging to you at all, though—does it feel like you've almost completed a cleanse? What foods do you miss, or what foods are you surprised that you *don't* miss?

Here's your menu for today:

Day Three Menu

Breakfast Blueberry-Banana Chia Pudding

Lunch Caesar Salad with Chunky Olive Tapenade

Dinner Roasted Kale & Cauliflower with Curry Cream

Dessert Whipped Cherry-Banana Freeze

The Blueberry-Banana Chia Pudding you'll be eating at breakfast will fill you up without weighing you down. Your gorgeous Caesar Salad with Chunky Olive Tapenade at lunch is packed with healthy, satisfying fats to fuel you through the afternoon. Roasted Kale & Cauliflower with Curry Cream makes a warm and warmly spiced dinner, and you'll end the day – and the cleanse – with a bowl of low-fat Whipped Cherry-Banana Freeze.

Nutritionally, today gives you middle-of-the-road amounts of fat and protein plus tons of filling fiber and plenty of energy-lending carbs.

Nutritional Totals for Day 3:
1425 calories | 52 grams fat | 228 grams carbohydrates
59 grams fiber | 46 grams protein | 980 milligrams sodium

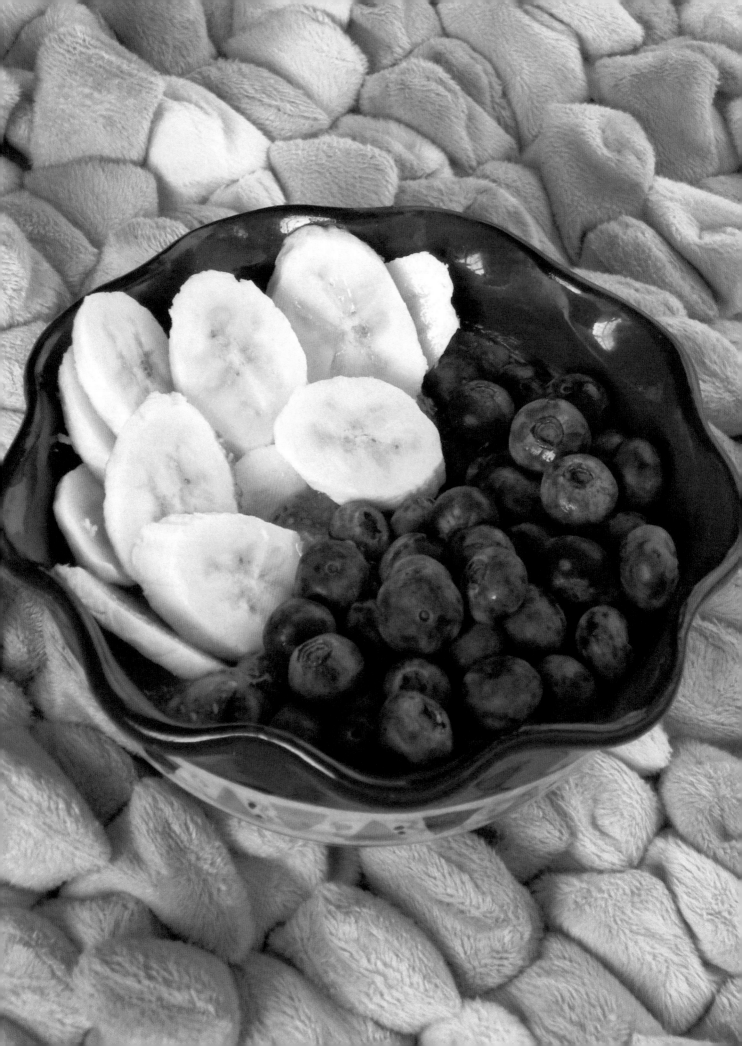

Blueberry-Banana Chia Pudding

When you add nutritious chia seeds to liquid, they form a tapioca-pudding-like gel that's rich in fiber and protein. Fresh fruit provides sweetness, but if the berries and banana don't add enough flavor for you, finely mince one pitted Medjool date and stir it into the pudding with the blueberries. You can also feel free to make this with nondairy milk in place of the water—coconut and hempseed milk are great nut-free options, or you can use almond milk if you don't mind including nuts in your cleanse.

2 tablespoons chia seeds
2/3 cup lukewarm water
1 large, very ripe banana, peeled and sliced
¾ cup fresh blueberries
Ground cinnamon, for sprinkling (optional)

Either the night before or 30 minutes before breakfast, combine the chia seeds and water in a medium bowl and stir together. Either refrigerate overnight, or set aside on the countertop for 30 minutes. The next morning (or 30 minutes later), stir the chia seed mixture. It should have thickened up significantly. Add half the banana slices to the chia seed gel and use a fork to mash them up into a pudding. Top the pudding with the remaining banana slices and the blueberries. Sprinkle with cinnamon, if desired, and serve immediately.

Nutritional Information:
305 calories, 10 grams fat, 54.9 grams carbs, 6 grams protein

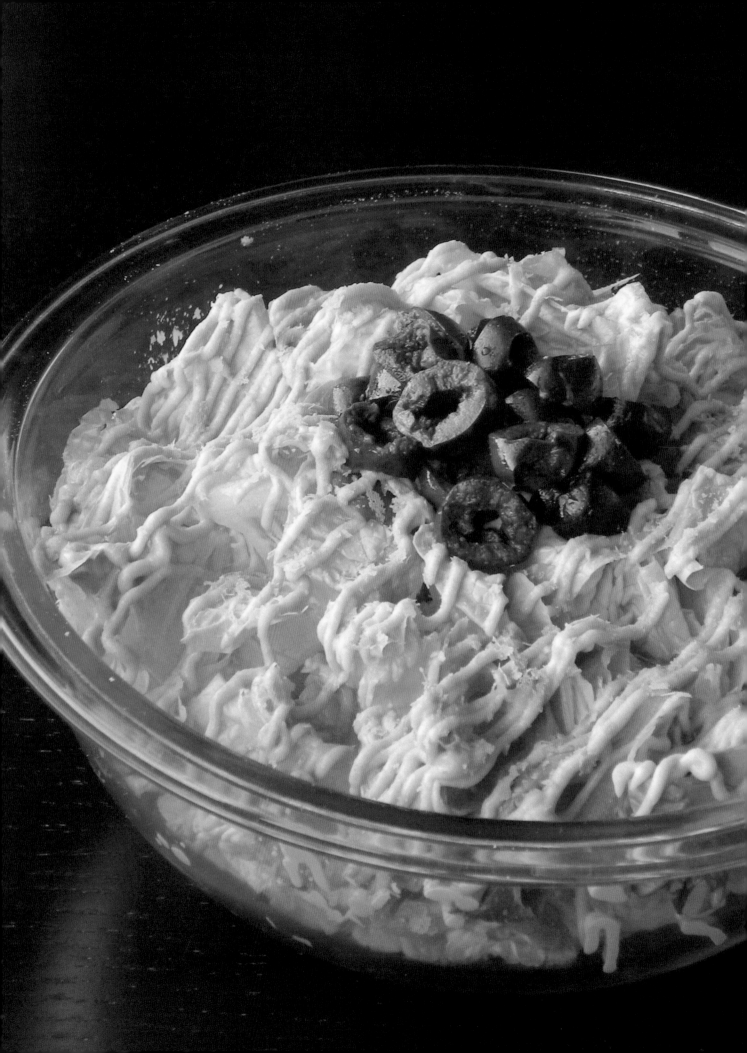

Caesar Salad with Chunky Olive Tapenade

Now this, my friends, is what I call a salad. There will be no daintily dipping your fork in a meager tablespoon or two of thin dressing here—this recipe makes a generous serving of thick, rich, creamy avocado dressing, and you get to eat the whole portion, plus a scoop of salty olive tapenade, atop a huge bed of crisp romaine. Heavenly! (Note: Not into olives? No big deal—just leave them out, or even replace them with a tablespoon of raw sunflower seeds for crunch.)

1 medium ripe avocado, pitted, peeled, and chopped
3 to 4 tablespoons water
2 tablespoons nutritional yeast
2 tablespoons fresh lemon juice
1 small clove garlic, peeled and minced (optional)

¼ teaspoon sea salt
1 (5-oz.) bag chopped romaine lettuce
¼ cup Kalamata olives, coarsely chopped
Additional nutritional yeast, for sprinkling (optional)

If you already prepared and set aside all the components last night, skip to step 3.

If you did not already prepare the dressing last night, combine the chopped avocado, 3 tablespoons water, nutritional yeast, lemon juice, garlic (if desired), and sea salt in a food processor (a mini processor works well here). Blend until completely smooth, adding another tablespoon of water if needed. Add the entire bag of romaine lettuce to a large bowl. Drizzle the whole batch of avocado dressing on top and toss lightly to combine. Top with the chopped olives and additional nutritional yeast, if desired.

Nutritional Information:
377 calories, 28.9 grams fat, 28.2 grams carbs, 12.1 grams protein

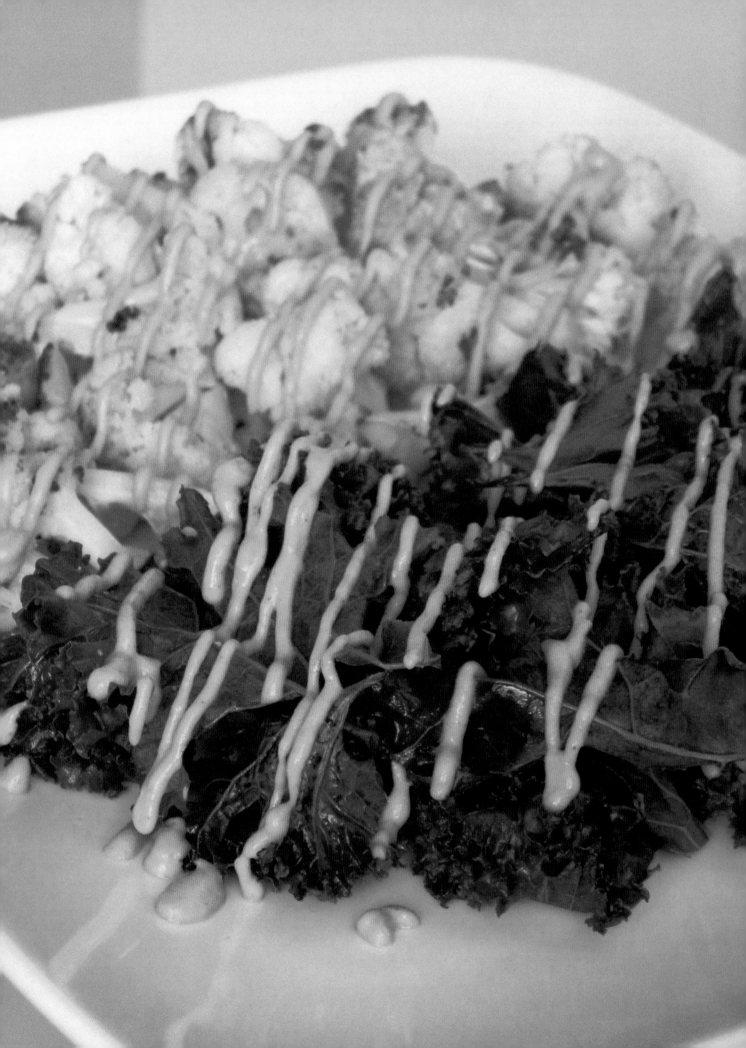

Roasted Kale & Cauliflower with Curry Cream

This dinner has four awesome things all on one plate: cauliflower, kale, chickpeas, and curry! It might just be my favorite meal on the whole cleanse.

1 small head cauliflower, stemmed and cut into florets
1/3 cup chickpeas, rinsed and drained
3 tablespoons water
2 tablespoons nutritional yeast
1 tablespoon tahini

1 tablespoon lemon juice
1½ teaspoons curry powder
½ teaspoon prepared yellow mustard
¼ teaspoon sea salt
1 small bunch kale, stems removed, leaves torn into bite-size pieces

About 45 minutes to an hour before dinner, preheat the oven to 425°F and line a baking sheet with parchment paper or a nonstick silicone mat.

While the oven is heating up, cut your cauliflower into medium florets and spread them evenly across the baking sheet. (If you like, you may mist the cauliflower lightly with cooking spray and sprinkle it with a couple pinches of salt. Cooking spray is an oil, and is not technically not permitted on the cleanse, but a very light coating will help roast the sugars in the cauliflower. This is completely optional, though.)

Place the cauliflower in the preheated oven and bake for 15 minutes.

Meanwhile, make the curry cream sauce by combining the chickpeas, water, nutritional yeast, tahini, lemon juice, curry powder, mustard, and salt in a blender or food processor and blending until smooth.

Remove the pan from the oven and carefully flip and stir the cauliflower around. Return to the oven for 10 more minutes.

Meanwhile, de-stem the kale and tear the leaves into large pieces. After the ten-minute timer goes off, remove the pan from the oven again. Stir the cauliflower around and scoot it all over to one-third to one-half of the baking sheet (it's okay to pile it up a little). Spread the kale across the now-open one-half to two-thirds of the baking sheet. (At this point, you may also mist the kale with cooking spray and sprinkle with a pinch of salt, but again, this is optional.)

Return the pan to the oven and roast for 5 more minutes, until the edges of some of the kale leaves have just begun to crisp up. Remove from the oven and let cool for 2-3 minutes before serving.

Dollop or drizzle the curry cream sauce over the hot roasted kale and cauliflower, and enjoy!

Nutritional Information:
424 calories, 12.6 grams fat, 66.2 grams carbs, 25.7 grams protein

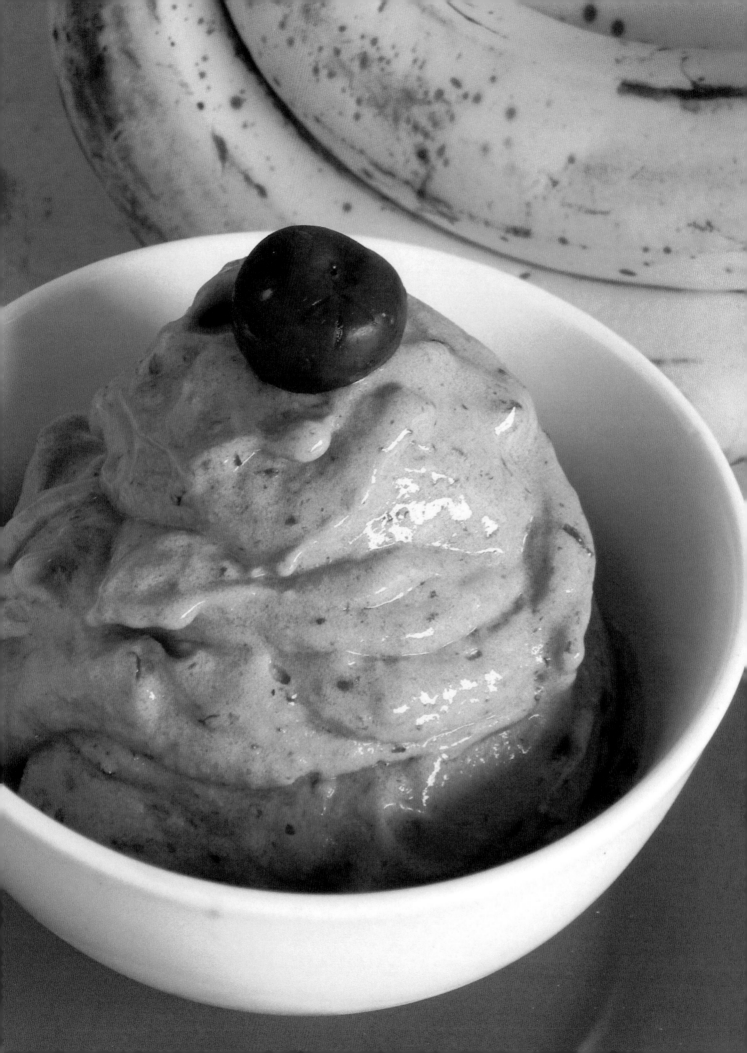

Whipped Cherry Banana Freeze

Frozen bananas make the perfect base for "instant" soft-serve ice cream. Cherries add sweetness and antioxidants to this low-fat dessert.

2 small (or 1½ large), very ripe bananas, peeled,
    sliced, and frozen overnight
½ (10-oz.) bag frozen cherries

Remove the sliced bananas and the cherries from the freezer about 5 minutes before you plan to make dessert.

When ready, place the sliced bananas and cherries into the bowl of a food processor. Pulse several times, until they begin to break down, and then process until completely smooth and whipped, stopping every 30 seconds or so to scrape down the sides and help the mixture get moving. It may take several minutes, but be patient—it will smooth out, and the result will be a lovely ice-cream-like consistency.

Serve immediately!

Nutritional Information:
319 calories, 0.8 grams fat, 78.3 grams carbs, 1.8 grams protein

post-cleanse guidelines

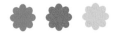

*C*ongratulations—you did it! You completed The REAL FOOD Cleanse, and I'm betting you breezed through it with flying colors!

How do you feel? Did you lose some weight? Do you feel lighter, happier, or more energetic? Are you sleeping a little more soundly at night? Is your digestion humming along smoothly now? No matter what your results have been, I'm sure you want to keep cruising along in your weight/energy/mood/sleep/digestion improvements now that you've gotten off to such a great start.

The first question on your lips is probably "What do I do/eat now?" While the answer is quite broad, as every body is different, here is my advice for how to reincorporate certain foods and re-diversify your diet but keep your new healthy lifestyle habits going strong.

Step 1: Continue basing your diet around the foods you ate during the cleanse.
Raw and cooked vegetables, fresh fruits, beans, and healthy fat sources (like tahini, coconut, and avocado) are items you should continue to include in your diet every single day. The easiest way to do this is to enjoy fruit at breakfast, a big portion of raw vegetables at lunch (for example, as large salads or crudités platters), cooked veggies and beans at dinner, and fruit-based desserts/treats—just like you have been all throughout the cleanse! You'll start adding back other foods in addition to these "green light foods" (see page 53), but keep these staples as the basis of your diet.

Step 2: Add back other "green light foods" (see page 53), slowly.
There are some foods that were not included in the cleanse but which you can now welcome back into your diet, such as gluten-free whole grains and healthful oils. Take it easy on these additions: keep serving size in mind (about ¾ cup cooked grains and/or 1 tablespoon oil at a time) and don't eat these foods at every single meal right off the bat.

Step 3: Add back "yellow light foods" (see page 53), one at a time and with caution.
"Yellow light foods" are foods that are either potentially irritating/allergenic or should simply be consumed mindfully and in moderation. Add back only one type of food from this list at

a time, no more frequently than every other day, beginning the day after your cleanse ends.

For example, the first day after your cleanse, you could enjoy some organic tempeh – a soy product – but have nothing else from this "yellow light" list. You're free to have organic soy the following (second) day as well, but again, nothing else from this list. Then, the next (third) day, you might add back nuts by snacking on ¼ cup of raw pecans in the afternoon. For that day and the following day, you are allowed to have both soy and nuts (though you don't have to have both), but nothing else from this list. Carry on in this fashion, adding one "yellow light" food type every other day, until you've added back everything you care to resume eating.

Pay close attention to how your body reacts to each one of these food additions—if you no-tice clear negative sensations (such as GI distress or stomach pain, diarrhea, headaches or body aches, unusual fatigue, etc.) within 48 hours of eating any of these items, it is probably something you will want to keep out of your diet for good. Be especially attentive if/when adding back gluten-containing grains or grain products—many folks are sensitive to gluten but don't realize it!

Step 4: Avoid "red light foods" (see page 54)—but don't let it rule your life.
"Red light foods" are things that, for all intents and purposes, I recommend you don't eat. That said, there's really no such thing as "never," is there? Life happens, and we'll inevitably find ourselves having a bite of a friend's birthday cake, or eating the croutons that came on our restaurant salad, or resorting to a packet of instant oatmeal at a hotel breakfast. So I say roll with the punches—don't knowingly eat these foods if you can avoid it, and certainly don't seek them out, but if a bite or two sneaks into your diet every now and then, it's not the end of the world. Besides, you'll be eating so healthfully all the rest of the time that your body will have no problem disposing of a morsel of junk every once in a great while. Life goes on!

Green Light Foods

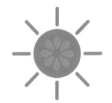

Any and all vegetables, raw and cooked

Fresh fruits

Dried fruit, in moderation

Beans and lentils

Avocados

Tahini

Seeds: sunflower, pumpkin, sesame, chia, flax, hemp

Coconut butter and milk and unsweetened shredded coconut

Gluten-free whole grains: quinoa, brown rice, millet, gluten-free oats, etc.

Healthy cold-pressed oils: coconut oil, extra-virgin olive oil

Green, white, oolong and herbal tes

Nutritional Yeast

Sea salt, herbs, and spices

Stevia

Yellow Light Foods

Organic soy foods: tempeh, tofu, edamame, tamari/soy sauce

Other whole-grain products, such as breads and pastas (preferably no more
than 1-2 servings per day), either gluten-containing or gluten-free

Nuts and nut butters: almonds, Brazil nuts, cashews, hazelnuts, macadamia nuts, pecans, pine nuts,
pistacthios, walnuts and their butters

Organic peanuts and/or peanut butter

Healthier forms of chocolate: cocoa/cacao powder, dark or raw chocolate bars

Coffee and black tea, in small amounts (1 cup per day is fine)

Unrefined sweeteners: maple syrup, coconut nectar, palm sugar, date sugar, evaporated cane juice,
etc. (in small quanitites; sweeten with whole dates when possible!)

Alcohol, on occasion, in reasonable quantities

Milk and other dairy products (butter, ghee, yogurt, kefir, cheese, etc.) from pasture-raised, grass-fed
cows, goats, or sheep* (or nondairy alternatives), as desired

100% pasture-raised, grass-fed meat/poultry/eggs* and/or wild-caught fish and other seafood, if
desired

*Check out www.eatwild.com to find properly-raised and sustainably-produced animal products from farms
near you.

Red Light Foods

Processed junk foods—if you're wondering whether something is considered

junk food, it probably is! If the label lists more than 5-7 ingredients (especially if many of them are

unrecognizable), don't buy or eat it.

Refined (white) flours and grains

Refined sugars (white sugar, brown sugar, high-fructose corn syrup, etc.)

Processed vegetable oils and hydrogenated fats

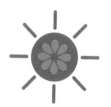

Artificial sweeteners (aspartame, Splenda, etc.)

Pop/soda, regular OR diet

Conventional, industrially-produced dairy products

Factory-farmed meat, poultry, eggs, and fish

frequently asked **questions**

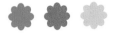

When am I supposed to eat each meal?

It's completely up to you! Everyone has a different schedule, so you're the best judge of what'll work for you. As for dessert, you can eat it whenever you like—most cleansers enjoy it either after dinner or as an afternoon snack.

Do I have to buy everything organic?

Choosing organic foods whenever possible can reduce your exposure to the pesticides, chemical additives, and genetically modified organisms (GMOs) often present in conventionally grown food products. That said, if you're working with a limited budget, buying organic is completely optional. If you'd like to be selective in your organic food shopping, my personal recommendation for this cleanse is to choose organic versions of the fresh fruits and vegetables that you'll be eating or using without peeling, such as the berries, cherries, apple, cucumber, bell pepper, baby carrots, and all the leafy greens called for.

What is coconut butter? Is it different from coconut oil?

Yes, very different! Coconut *oil* is the pure fat that's extracted from the coconut meat, while coconut *butter* IS the coconut meat, dried and ground into a smooth paste. Think of the difference between peanut oil and peanut butter—same idea. Oils aren't permitted on the cleanse, so definitely seek out coconut *butter*, or replace it with almond butter or tahini.

If I can't have my morning coffee, what am I supposed to drink in the a.m.?

You're welcome to drink green tea, white tea, oolong tea, herbal tea, or hot water with a splash of lemon juice. Green, white, and oolong teas do contain some caffeine, which technically isn't allowed during the cleanse, but if you're accustomed to downing several cups of coffee a day, it's perfectly acceptable to transition to tea instead of going caffeine-free cold-turkey. Being a coffee lover myself, I know it can be frustrating to give it up, even for just a few days, but oftentimes simply having something else hot to drink in its place can be a big help.

Can I use stevia while on the cleanse?

I'd prefer you didn't. Omitting added sweeteners from your diet – even an all-natural, calorie-free, zero-glycemic sweetener like stevia – is a key step in getting back in touch with the natural flavors of whole foods and readjusting your taste buds to expect less added sweetness in your diet. It's only three days—try your very best to put the stevia away for just 72 hours and see how you do. You can always bring it back into your diet on day 4! You might even find yourself using a little less of it than you did before the cleanse.

If you want to add sweetness to something (like any of the breakfasts or desserts), add one very finely minced, pitted Medjool date. Then you're getting fiber and minerals along with the natural sugars! As far as tea, etc. try your very best to drink it plain for the three days of the cleanse. If you absolutely must have that hot drink and you must add a tiny touch of sweetness, then use ONLY 5-7 droplets of liquid stevia (not the stevia in packets, which also contain fillers like maltodextrin or silica) and no more, once per day. But I do urge you to challenge yourself to try, for just these three days, to go sweetener-free. You can do it!

What if I'm simply starving and I HAVE to have a snack at some point?

Have a handful of baby carrots. You purchased a small bag, but are only using ¾ cup of them at lunch on day 2, so the remainder of the bag can be your emergency snack stash for the duration of the cleanse. Beyond that, if you feel you must have additional snacks, you may want to transition to the "Bulk It Up" version of the plan (see page 18 for details), or at least add a handful of sunflower seeds or another banana to each day for some extra calories.

I'm experiencing gas/bloating/stomach discomfort/bowel changes. Is this normal?

Yes, it's not unusual. You're consuming a great deal of dietary fiber (both soluble and insoluble) on this cleanse, which can be a bit of a shock to the system if you're not accustomed to it. Fiber benefits us in countless ways, from regulating bowel motility to binding and eliminating toxins released during the cleanse. The discomfort shouldn't last long, so hang in there!

If you've had trouble digesting beans in the past, and you feel it's the beans that are causing you trouble, I strongly recommend you try Eden brand canned beans—they cook their beans with kombu, a Japanese sea vegetable that helps make the beans more easily digestible.

I want to cleanse longer than just 3 days. Can I do The REAL FOOD Cleanse multiple times in a row?

Sure! You can definitely do two back-to-back rounds of the cleanse (which makes for easy shopping; just double all the items on the Shopping List), or even an "expanded" version where you make double of every recipe and do each day twice in a row (e.g. Day 1 – Day 1 – Day 2 – Day 2 – Day 3 – Day 3). After two rounds in a row, I'd like you to take at least a one-day break where you spike your calories a bit, but still eat very healthfully—just increase your portion sizes a tad or add a couple snacks (see the Bulk It Up plan on page 18 for ideas). Adding a higher-calorie day every now and then helps "remind" your metabolism not to slow down too much, which can happen with long-term low-calorie dieting.

Now that my cleanse is over, I have no idea what to eat/cook/make. Help!

Never fear! First, high-tail it over to my website, chefambershea.com, for oodles of free healthy recipes. You can even subscribe to receive new posts by email so you never miss a post! The next step will be picking up copies of my cookbooks, *Practically Raw* and *Practically Raw Desserts*, which are jam-packed with fresh, vibrant, unprocessed, health-promoting recipes (over 240 in both books combined) that can be made 100% raw or cooked/baked for added variety and flexibility. Finally, I urge you to come join The REAL FOOD Cleanse Facebook group (see next question), where you can seek specific recipes, ask for additional cookbook recommendations, and/or generally benefit from the wisdom and experience of other cleansers!

I have another question that you didn't answer! What do I do?

Good news—when you purchased this ebook, you also earned free access to The REAL FOOD Cleanse Facebook group. This is a private forum on Facebook where both current and past cleansers can swap tips and experiences, share ideas, ask questions, give advice, and provide each other with motivation and support. I myself check in often to answer your questions directly as well. Join us at:

http://www.facebook.com/groups/TheREALFOODCleanse/

conclusion

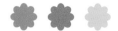

Now that you're armed with the tools and knowledge you need to keep your new healthy lifestyle rolling forward, I have every confidence that a happier, sexier, livelier, and longer-lived YOU is right around the corner. Keep chasing that strong, beautiful, and capable person, and don't ever stop. You are worth it.

To your health!

Amber

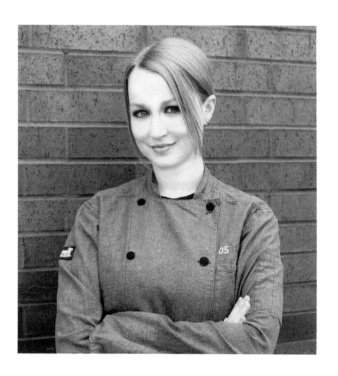

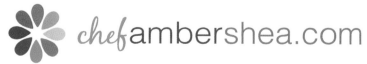

Also by Amber Shea Crawley ...

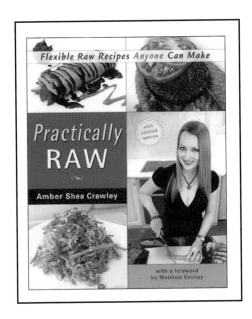

Practically Raw: Flexible Raw Recipes Anyone Can Make

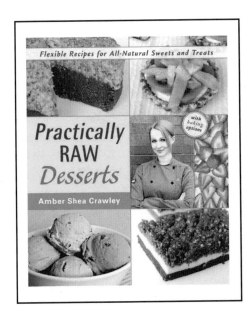

Practically Raw Desserts: Flexible Recipes For
All-Natural Sweets and Treats